My Fit & Healthy Dash Diet Slow Cooker Cooking Plan

Lose Weight with These Tasteful Recipes

Carmela Rojas

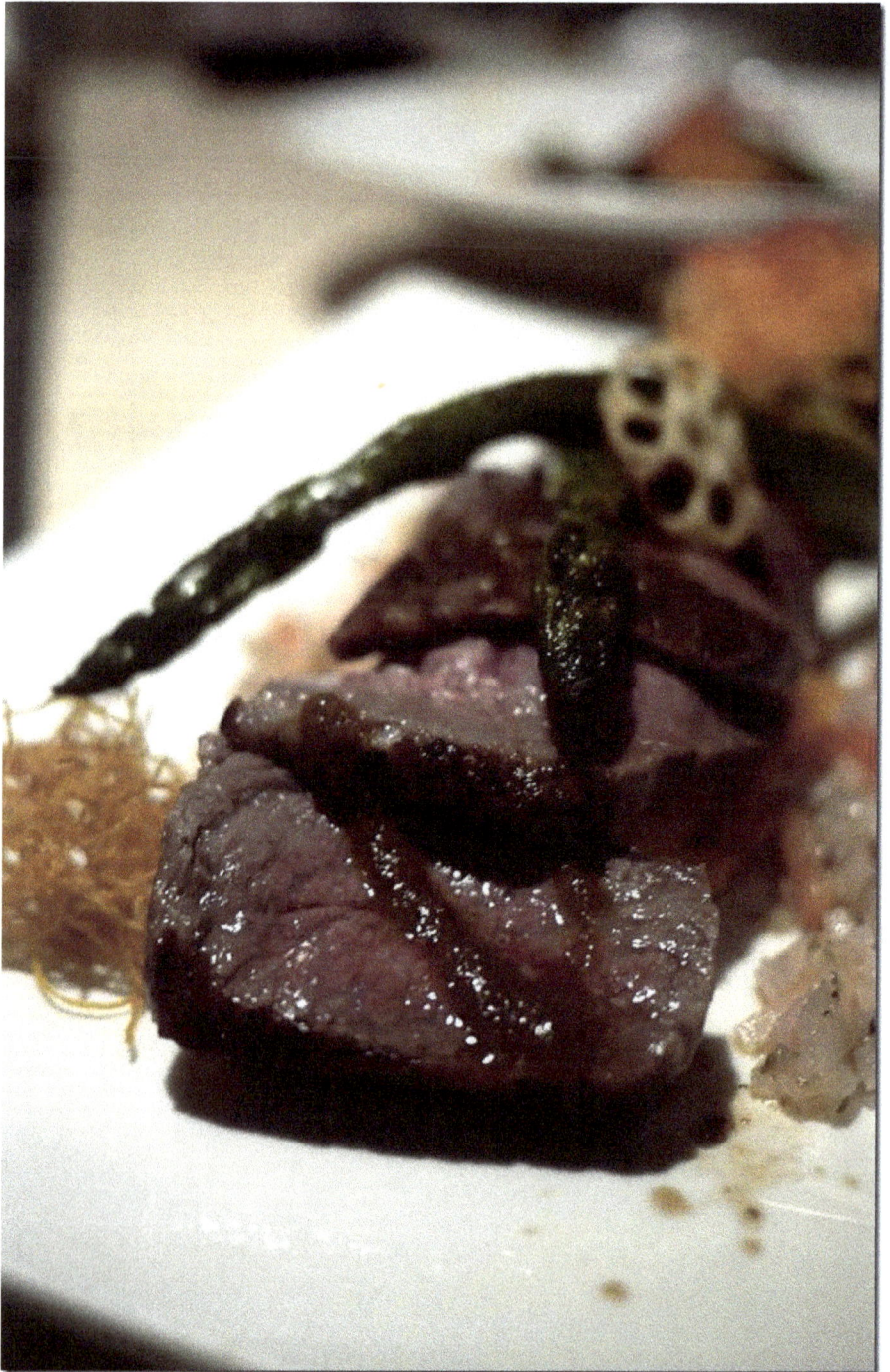

TABLE OF CONTENTS

Smoky Beef Roast

Servings: 8 Servings

Ingredients:

- 2 pounds (900 g) beef round roast
- 8 ounces (255 g) mushrooms, sliced
- ½ cup (80 g) sliced onion
- ½ teaspoon minced garlic
- 1½ cups (355 ml) coffee
- 1 teaspoon liquid smoke
- ½ teaspoon chili powder
- ½ teaspoon black pepper

Directions:

1. Place roast in slow cooker. Combine remaining ingredients and pour over roast. Cover and cook on low for 9 to 10 hours.

Nutrition Info:

Per serving: 162 g water; 157 calories (25% from fat, 69% from protein, 6% from carb); 26 g protein; 4 g total fat; 1 g saturated fat; 2 g monounsaturated fat; 0 g polyunsaturated fat; 2 g carb; 1 g fiber; 1 g sugar; 275 mg phosphorus; 29 mg calcium; 2 mg iron;

74 mg sodium; 550 mg potassium; 47 IU vitamin A; 0 mg ATE vitamin E; 2 mg vitamin C; 57 mg cholesterol

Fajitas

Servings: 6 Servings

Ingredients:

- 1½ pounds (680 g) flank steak
- 1 can (14 ounces, or 400 g) no-salt-added diced tomatoes, undrained
- 1 jalapeño, seeded and chopped
- ½ teaspoon minced garlic
- 1 teaspoon coriander
- 1 teaspoon cumin
- 1 teaspoon chili powder
- 2 cups (320 g) sliced onion
- 2 cups (300 g) sliced green bell pepper
- 2 cups (300 g) sliced red bell pepper
- 1 tablespoon (1 g) fresh cilantro

Directions:

1. Thinly slice steak across the grain into strips; place in slow cooker. Add tomatoes, jalapeño, garlic, coriander, cumin, and chili powder. Cover and cook on low for 7 hours. Add onion, peppers, and cilantro.

Cover and cook 1 to 2 hours longer or until meat is tender.

Nutrition Info:

Per serving: 278 g water; 279 calories (32% from fat, 48% from protein, 19% from carb); 34 g protein; 10 g total fat; 4 g saturated fat; 4 g monounsaturated fat; 1 g polyunsaturated fat; 14 g carb; 4 g fiber; 7 g sugar; 295 mg phosphorus; 65 mg calcium; 4 mg iron; 83 mg sodium; 804 mg potassium; 1999 IU vitamin A; 0 mg ATE vitamin E; 116 mg vitamin C; 62 mg cholesterol

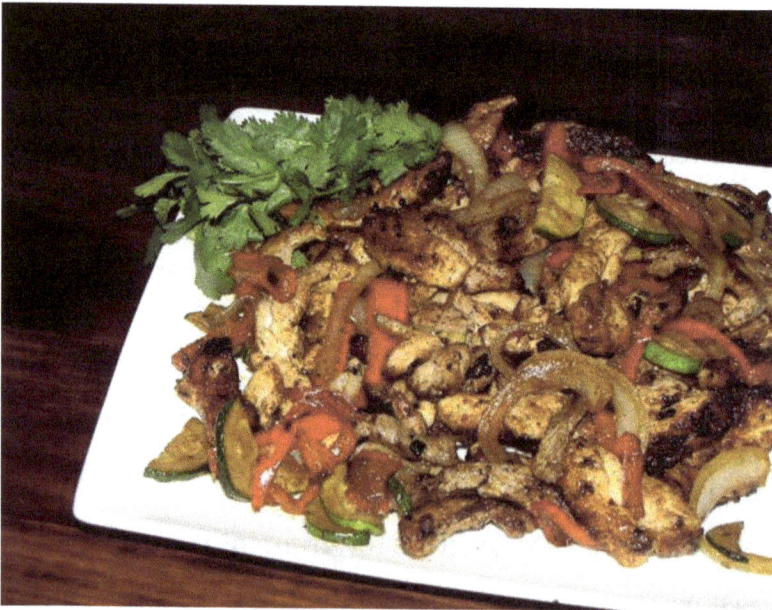

Pork With Squash And Apples

Servings: About 4

Cooking Time: 6 Hrs 15 Mins

Ingredients:

- 4 boneless Pork Chops
- Ground Black Pepper
- 1 sliced Onion
- 2 tsp. Olive Oil
- 1 minced clove Garlic
- 1 sliced Red Bell Pepper
- ½ tsp. ground Cumin
- ½ tsp. ground Cinnamon
- ½ cup Chicken Broth
- ½ cup Coconut Milk
- 1 diced tart Apple
- 1 cup cubed Squash
- 2 tbsp. chopped Parsley

Directions:

1. Sauté the pork chops in oil for 6 mins.
2. Transfer them to slow cooker.

3. In same pan, , sauté rest of the ingredients except apple, broth, squash and coconut milk.
4. Pour the mixture into the slow cooker.
5. Now, add the rest of the ingredients.
6. Cook on "low" for 6 hrs.
7. Serve the Pork chops on heated plates after garnishing with parsley.

Nutrition Info:

(Estimated Amount Per Serving): 322 Calories; 25 g Total Fat; 74 mg Cholesterol; 350 mg Sodium; 10 mg Carbohydrates; 3 g Dietary Fiber; 19 g Protein

Hawaiian Steak

Servings: 5 Servings

Ingredients:

- 1 pound (455 g) flank steak
- Dash black pepper
- 30 ounces (840 g) fruit cocktail, canned in syrup
- 1 tablespoon (15 ml) olive oil
- 1 tablespoon (15 ml) lemon juice
- ¼ cup (60 ml) low-sodium teriyaki sauce
- 1 teaspoon red wine vinegar
- ½ teaspoons minced garlic

Directions:

1. Place flank steak in slow cooker. Sprinkle with pepper. Drain fruit cocktail, reserving ¼ cup (60 ml) syrup. Combine reserved syrup with remaining ingredients, except fruit. Pour syrup mixture over steak. Cover and cook on low 7 to 9 hours. Add drained fruit during the last 10 minutes of cooking time. Cut meat into thin slices across the grain to serve.

Nutrition Info:

Per serving: 220 g water; 296 calories (33% from fat, 35% from protein, 32% from carb); 26 g protein; 11 g total fat; 4 g saturated fat; 5 g monounsaturated fat; 1 g polyunsaturated fat; 24 g carb; 2 g fiber; 21 g sugar; 219 mg phosphorus; 29 mg calcium; 2 mg iron; 90 mg sodium; 480 mg potassium; 519 IU vitamin A; 0 mg ATE vitamin E; 6 mg vitamin C; 50 mg cholesterol

Creamy Steak

Servings: 6 Servings

Ingredients:

- 1½ pounds (680 g) beef round steak
- ¼ cup (31 g) flour
- 2 tablespoons (28 ml) olive oil
- 1½ cups (240 g) thickly sliced onions
- 1 cup (150 g) green bell pepper strips
- 10 ounces (280 g) low-sodium cream of mushroom soup

Directions:

1. Cut steak into serving-size pieces. Dredge in flour. Heat oil in a nonstick skillet and brown the steak on both sides. Place browned steak in slow cooker. Top with onion and pepper slices. Pour soup over all, making sure steak pieces are covered. Cover and cook on low 4 to 5 hours.

Nutrition Info:

Per serving: 182 g water; 248 calories (34% from fat, 45% from protein, 21% from carb); 28 g protein; 9 g total fat; 2 g saturated

fat; 5 g monounsaturated fat; 1 g polyunsaturated fat; 13 g carb; 2 g fiber; 3 g sugar; 295 mg phosphorus; 22 mg calcium; 3 mg iron; 77 mg sodium; 719 mg potassium; 96 IU vitamin A; 1 mg ATE vitamin E; 23 mg vitamin C; 66 mg cholesterol

Asian Pot Roast

Servings: 8 Servings

Ingredients:

- 3 pounds (1 1/3 kg) beef chuck roast
- 2 tablespoons (16 g) flour
- 1 tablespoon (15 ml) olive oil
- 1 cup (160 g) chopped onion
- ¼ teaspoon pepper
- ½ cup (120 ml) low-sodium soy sauce
- 1 cup (235 ml) water
- ½ teaspoon ground ginger

Directions:

1. Dredge roast in flour. Heat oil in a skillet over medium-high heat and brown roast on both sides. Place in slow cooker. Top with onions and pepper. Combine soy sauce, water, and ginger. Pour over meat. Cover and cook on high 30 minutes. Reduce heat to low and cook 8 to 10 hours. Slice and serve with rice.

Nutrition Info:

Per serving: 159 g water; 396 calories (35% from fat, 60% from protein, 5% from carb); 57 g protein; 15 g total fat; 5 g saturated fat; 7 g monounsaturated fat; 1 g polyunsaturated fat; 5 g carb; 1 g fiber; 1 g sugar; 482 mg phosphorus; 24 mg calcium; 7 mg iron; 164 mg sodium; 554 mg potassium; 4 IU vitamin A; 0 mg ATE vitamin E; 2 mg vitamin C; 172 mg cholesterol

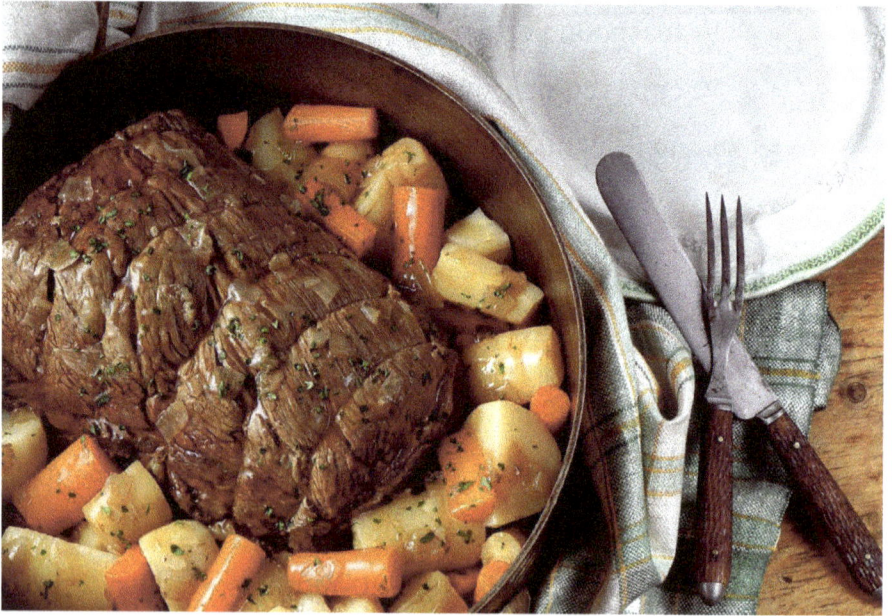

Slow Cooker Shredded Pork

Servings: 8 Servings

Ingredients:

- 4 pounds (1.8 kg) pork shoulder roast
- 1½ teaspoons minced garlic
- 1 cup (160 g) finely chopped onion
- 4 ounces (115 g) diced green chilies
- 1 cup (235 ml) cider vinegar

Directions:

1. Place roast in slow cooker. Combine remaining ingredients and pour over roast. Cover and cook on low 8 to 10 hours. Remove to a cutting board and shred with two forks, discarding fat and bones.

Nutrition Info:

Per serving: 206 g water; 550 calories (69% from fat, 29% from protein, 2% from carb); 39 g protein; 41 g total fat; 14 g saturated fat; 18 g monounsaturated fat; 4 g polyunsaturated fat; 2 g carb; 0 g fiber; 1 g sugar; 422 mg phosphorus; 42 mg calcium; 2 mg iron; 150 mg sodium; 738 mg potassium; 16 IU vitamin A; 5 mg ATE vitamin E; 3 mg vitamin C; 161 mg cholesterol

Beef Brisket

Servings: About 12

Cooking Time: 8 Hrs

Ingredients:

- 5 pounds Beef Brisket (trimmed)
- 2 minced cloves Garlic
- ½ tsp. Black Pepper
- 2 tbsp. Brown Sugar
- 2 tsp. Paprika (smoked)
- 2 sliced Onions
- 1 ½ cup Beef Broth
- 3 diced Carrots
- 3 sliced Parsnips
- 14 ounces diced Tomatoes

Directions:

1. In a bowl, mix paprika, brown sugar, black pepper and garlic.
2. Coat beef with paprika mixture and place it into the slow cooker.
3. Now, place all the remaining ingredients in layers.
4. Cook on "low" for 8 hrs.

5. Transfer the beef to a cutting board.

6. Leave it for 10 mins at least.

7. Slice and serve with the cooked vegetables.

Nutrition Info:

(Estimated Amount Per Serving): 283 Calories; 15 g Total Fat; 128 mg Cholesterol; 385 mg Sodium; 7 mg Carbohydrates; 2 g Dietary Fiber; 44 g Protein

Beef And Bacon In Beer

Servings: 6 Servings

Ingredients:

- 1½ pounds (680 g) beef stew meat, cubed
- 3 tablespoons (24 g) flour
- 4 tablespoons (60 ml) oil, divided
- 4 slices low-sodium bacon
- 1 cup (160 g) finely chopped onion
- 1 teaspoon minced garlic
- 1 teaspoon mustard
- 2 teaspoons no-salt-added tomato paste
- 2 cups (475 ml) beer, preferably dark
- 1 teaspoon low-sodium beef bouillon
- 1 teaspoon Worcestershire sauce
- ½ teaspoon sugar

Directions:

1. Toss the beef in the flour until covered. Heat 2 tablespoons (28 ml) of oil in a large frying pan or wok and fry the beef until brown. Remove the meat. In the remaining oil, gently fry the onion and the garlic until soft and transparent. Return the meat to the pan with

the onion and garlic. Add the remaining ingredients and cook until the sauce thickens. Put in the slow cooker and cook for approximately 7 hours or until tender.

Nutrition Info:

Per serving: 100 g water; 173 calories (67% from fat, 8% from protein, 25% from carb); 3 g protein; 11 g total fat; 2 g saturated fat; 3 g monounsaturated fat; 5 g polyunsaturated fat; 9 g carb; 1 g fiber; 2 g sugar; 55 mg phosphorus; 13 mg calcium; 0 mg iron; 138 mg sodium; 123 mg potassium; 32 IU vitamin A; 1 mg ATE vitamin E; 4 mg vitamin C; 6 mg cholesterol

Italian Swiss Steak

Servings: 6 Servings

Ingredients:

- 2 tablespoons (16 g) flour
- ¼ teaspoon black pepper
- 2 pounds (900 g) beef round steak
- 2 tablespoons (28 ml) olive oil
- 1 cup (160 g) sliced onion
- 1 can (8 ounces, or 225 g) no-salt-added tomato sauce
- 8 ounces (225 g) low-sodium spaghetti sauce
- ½ cup (120 ml) water
- ½ teaspoon basil
- ½ teaspoon oregano

Directions:

1. Combine flour and pepper in a resealable plastic bag. Cut steak into 6 pieces, add to bag, and shake to coat. Heat oil in a large skillet. Brown steak on both sides. Place onions in slow cooker. Place steak on top. Combine remaining ingredients and pour over steak. Cook on low 8 to 10 hours or on high 4 to 5 hours.

Nutrition Info:

Per serving: 214 g water; 308 calories (34% from fat, 48% from protein, 18% from carb); 36 g protein; 11 g total fat; 3 g saturated fat; 7 g monounsaturated fat; 1 g polyunsaturated fat; 13 g carb; 2 g fiber; 7 g sugar; 368 mg phosphorus; 31 mg calcium; 4 mg iron; 96 mg sodium; 911 mg potassium; 375 IU vitamin A; 0 mg ATE vitamin E; 11 mg vitamin C; 86 mg cholesterol

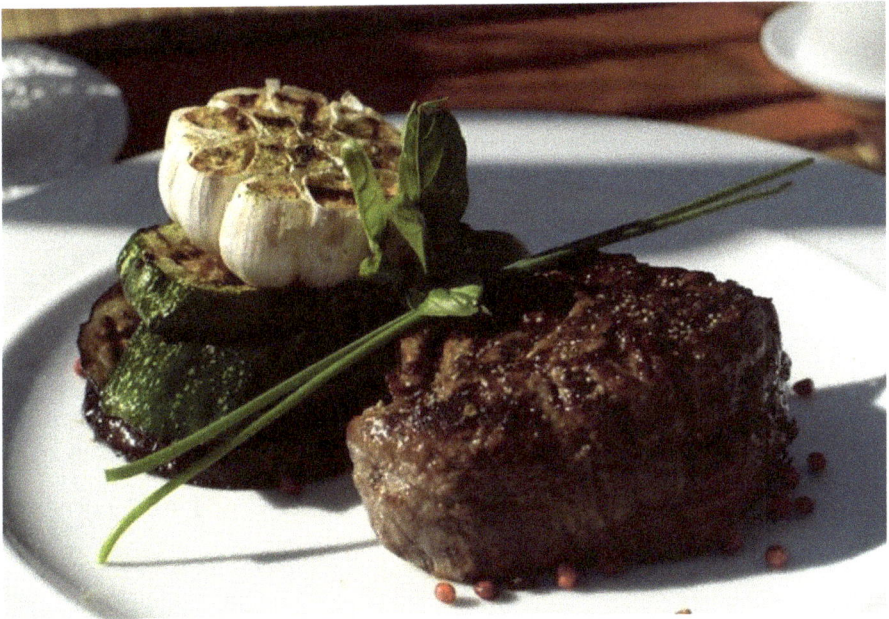

Green Beans With Smoked Sausage

Servings: 5 Servings

Ingredients:

- 1 pound (455 g) turkey smoked sausage, sliced ½–inch (1.3 cm) thick
- 1 pound (455 g) frozen green beans
- ½ cup (80 g) chopped onion
- ¼ cup (60 g) brown sugar

Directions:

1. Place sausage in slow cooker. Top with beans and then onion. Sprinkle with sugar. Cover and cook on low 4 to 5 hours.

Nutrition Info:

Per serving: 153 g water; 281 calories (50% from fat, 19% from protein, 31% from carb); 14 g protein; 16 g total fat; 6 g saturated fat; 8 g monounsaturated fat; 2 g polyunsaturated fat; 22 g carb; 3 g fiber; 13 g sugar; 42 mg phosphorus; 47 mg calcium; 2 mg iron; 626 mg sodium; 251 mg potassium; 626 IU vitamin A; 0 mg ATE vitamin E; 29 mg vitamin C; 64 mg cholesterol

Easy Swiss Steak

Servings: 6 Servings

Ingredients:

- 1 tablespoon (15 ml) vegetable oil
- ½ cup (60 g) flour
- ½ teaspoon black pepper
- ½ teaspoon paprika
- 2 pounds (900 g) round steak
- 2 cups (300 g) green bell pepper, sliced into rings
- 2 cups (300 g) red bell pepper, sliced into rings
- 4 cups (640 g) onion, sliced into rings
- 1 can (28 ounces, or 785 g) no-salt-added diced tomatoes

Directions:

1. Heat the oil in a skillet over medium heat. In a bowl, mix the flour, pepper, and paprika. Dredge the steaks in the flour mixture and place in the skillet. Brown steaks on both sides and remove from heat. In a slow cooker, alternate layers of steak, green pepper, red pepper, onion, and tomatoes. Cover and cook 6 to 8 hours on low until steaks are very tender.

Nutrition Info:

Per serving: 414 g water; 392 calories (22% from fat, 49% from protein, 29% from carb); 48 g protein; 9 g total fat; 3 g saturated fat; 3 g monounsaturated fat; 2 g polyunsaturated fat; 29 g carb; 5 g fiber; 11 g sugar; 366 mg phosphorus; 86 mg calcium; 6 mg iron; 83 mg sodium; 971 mg potassium; 1997 IU vitamin A; 0 mg ATE vitamin E; 124 mg vitamin C; 88 mg cholesterol

Easy Pepper Steak

Servings: 6 Servings

Ingredients:

- 1½ pounds (680 g) beef round steak
- ¼ cup (31 g) plus
- 1 tablespoon (8 g) flour, divided
- ¼ teaspoon pepper
- 1 cup (160 g) chopped or sliced onion
- ½ teaspoon minced garlic
- 1½ cups (225 g) green bell pepper, sliced in ½-inch (1.3 cm) strips
- 1 can (28 ounces, or 785 g) no-salt-added diced tomatoes
- 1 tablespoon (15 ml) low-sodium soy sauce
- 1 teaspoon Worcestershire sauce
- 3 tablespoons (45 ml) water

Directions:

1. Cut beef into strips. Combine ¼ cup (31 g) flour and pepper. Toss with beef until well coated. Place in slow cooker. Add onions, garlic, and green pepper slices. Mix well. Combine tomatoes, soy sauce, and

Worcestershire sauce. Pour into slow cooker. Cover and cook on low 8 to 10 hours. One hour before serving, turn to high. Combine remaining 1 tablespoon (8 g) flour and water to make smooth paste. Stir into slow cooker. Cover and cook until thickened. Serve over rice.

Nutrition Info:

Per serving: 275 g water; 211 calories (17% from fat, 54% from protein, 28% from carb); 28 g protein; 4 g total fat; 1 g saturated fat; 2 g monounsaturated fat; 0 g polyunsaturated fat; 15 g carb; 3 g fiber; 5 g sugar; 300 mg phosphorus; 56 mg calcium; 4 mg iron; 95 mg sodium; 807 mg potassium; 298 IU vitamin A; 0 mg ATE vitamin E; 46 mg vitamin C; 65 mg cholesterol

Sour Cream Pot Roast

Servings: 8 Servings

Ingredients:

- 4 pounds (1.8 kg) beef chuck roast
- 1 garlic clove, cut in half
- ½ teaspoon pepper
- ½ cup (65 g) chopped carrot
- ½ cup (50 g) chopped celery
- ½ cup (80 g) sliced onion
- ¾ cup (180 g) sour cream
- 3 tablespoons (24 g) flour
- ½ cup (120 ml) dry white wine

Directions:

1. Rub roast with garlic. Season with pepper. Place in slow cooker. Add carrots, celery, and onion. Combine sour cream, flour, and wine. Pour into slow cooker. Cover and cook on low 6 to 7 hours.

Nutrition Info:

Per serving: 186 g water; 538 calories (36% from fat, 60% from protein, 4% from carb); 76 g protein; 20 g total fat; 8 g saturated

fat; 8 g monounsaturated fat; 1 g polyunsaturated fat; 5 g carb; 1 g fiber; 1 g sugar; 642 mg phosphorus; 53 mg calcium; 9 mg iron; 171 mg sodium; 755 mg potassium; 1464 IU vitamin A; 23 mg ATE vitamin E; 2 mg vitamin C; 238 mg cholesterol

Beef With Italian Sauce

Servings: 10 Servings

Ingredients:

- 3 pounds (1 1/3 kg) beef round roast
- ¼ teaspoon garlic powder
- ¼ teaspoon pepper
- 4 ounces (115 g) mushrooms, sliced
- 1 cup (160 g) diced onion
- 14 ounces (390 g) low-sodium spaghetti sauce
- ½ cup (120 ml) low-sodium beef broth

Directions:

1. Cut roast in half. Combine garlic powder and pepper. Rub over both halves of the roast. Place in slow cooker. Top with mushrooms and onions. Combine spaghetti sauce and broth. Pour over roast. Cover and cook on low 8 to 9 hours. Slice roast. Serve in sauce over pasta.

Nutrition Info:

Per serving: 166 g water; 227 calories (28% from fat, 57% from protein, 15% from carb); 32 g protein; 7 g total fat; 2 g saturated fat; 3 g monounsaturated fat; 0 g polyunsaturated fat; 8 g carb; 2

g fiber; 5 g sugar; 326 mg phosphorus; 44 mg calcium; 3 mg iron; 105 mg sodium; 710 mg potassium; 246 IU vitamin A; 0 mg ATE vitamin E; 6 mg vitamin C; 68 mg cholesterol

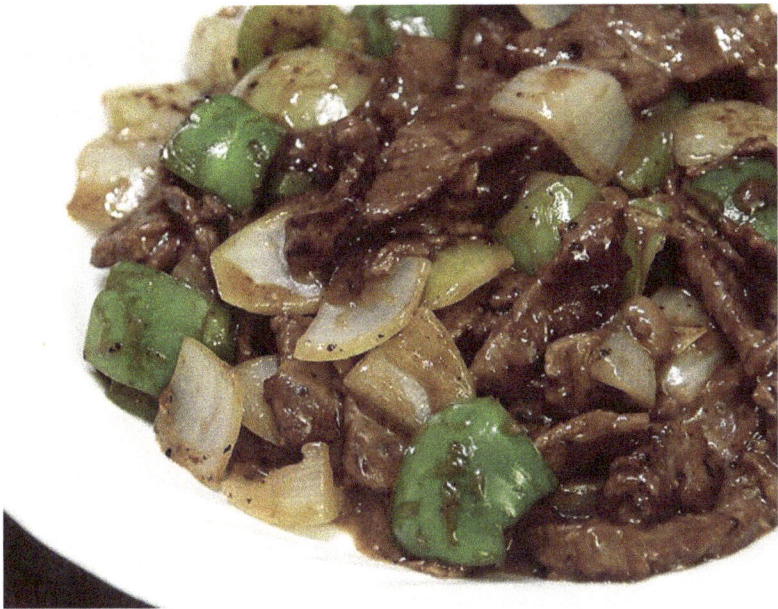

Mexican Steak Stew

Servings: 8 Servings

Ingredients:

- 2½ pounds (1.1 kg) beef round steak
- 1 cup (160 g) chopped onion
- 2 tablespoons (15 g) Salt-Free Mexican Seasoning
- 1 can (14 ounces, or 400 g) no-salt-added diced tomatoes, undrained
- 1 cup (150 g) red bell pepper, cut into 1-inch (2.5 cm) pieces

Directions:

1. Trim excess fat from beef and cut into 2-inch (5 cm) pieces. Combine with onion in slow cooker. Mix together seasoning and undrained tomatoes. Pour over beef. Place red pepper on top. Cover. Cook on low 6 to 8 hours or until beef is tender.

Nutrition Info:

Per serving: 183 g water; 201 calories (22% from fat, 68% from protein, 10% from carb); 33 g protein; 5 g total fat; 2 g saturated fat; 2 g monounsaturated fat; 0 g polyunsaturated fat; 5 g carb; 1

g fiber; 3 g sugar; 331 mg phosphorus; 26 mg calcium; 4 mg iron; 82 mg sodium; 705 mg potassium; 642 IU vitamin A; 0 mg ATE vitamin E; 30 mg vitamin C; 81 mg cholesterol

Beef And Beans

Servings: 8 Servings

Ingredients:

- 1½ pounds (680 g) beef round steak
- 1 tablespoon (11 g) mustard
- 1 tablespoon (7.5 g) chili powder
- ¼ teaspoon black pepper
- ½ teaspoon minced garlic
- 1 can (14 ounces, or 400 g) no-salt-added diced tomatoes
- 1 cup (160 g) chopped onion
- 2 cups (512 g) kidney beans

Directions:

1. Cut steak into thin strips. Combine mustard, chili powder, pepper, and garlic in a bowl. Add steak and toss to coat. Transfer to slow cooker. Add tomatoes and onion. Cover and cook on low 5 to 7 hours. Stir in beans. Cook 30 minutes longer.

Nutrition Info:

Per serving: 155 g water; 184 calories (16% from fat, 53% from protein, 31% from carb); 24 g protein; 3 g total fat; 1 g saturated fat; 1 g monounsaturated fat; 0 g polyunsaturated fat; 14 g carb; 5 g fiber; 2 g sugar; 268 mg phosphorus; 46 mg calcium; 4 mg iron; 63 mg sodium; 639 mg potassium; 339 IU vitamin A; 0 mg ATE vitamin E; 7 mg vitamin C; 48 mg cholesterol

Fajita Steak

Servings: 6 Servings

Ingredients:

- 1 can (14 ounces, or 400 g) no-salt-added diced tomatoes
- 4 ounces (115 g) diced green chilies
- ¼ cup (65 g) low-sodium salsa
- 1 can (8 ounces, or 225 g) no-salt-added tomato sauce
- 2 pounds (900 g) beef round steak, cut in 2-inch × 4-inch (5 cm × 10 cm) strips
- 2 tablespoons (14 g) Salt-Free Mexican Seasoning

Directions:

1. Combine all ingredients in slow cooker. Cover and cook on low 6 to 8 hours or until meat is tender but not overcooked. Check meat occasionally to make sure it isn't cooking dry. If it begins to look dry, stir in up to 1 cup (235 ml) water.

Nutrition Info:

Per serving: 231 g water; 224 calories (22% from fat, 66% from protein, 13% from carb); 36 g protein; 5 g total fat; 2 g saturated

fat; 2 g monounsaturated fat; 0 g polyunsaturated fat; 7 g carb; 2 g fiber; 4 g sugar; 361 mg phosphorus; 40 mg calcium; 4 mg iron; 191 mg sodium; 897 mg potassium; 264 IU vitamin A; 0 mg ATE vitamin E; 18 mg vitamin C; 86 mg cholesterol

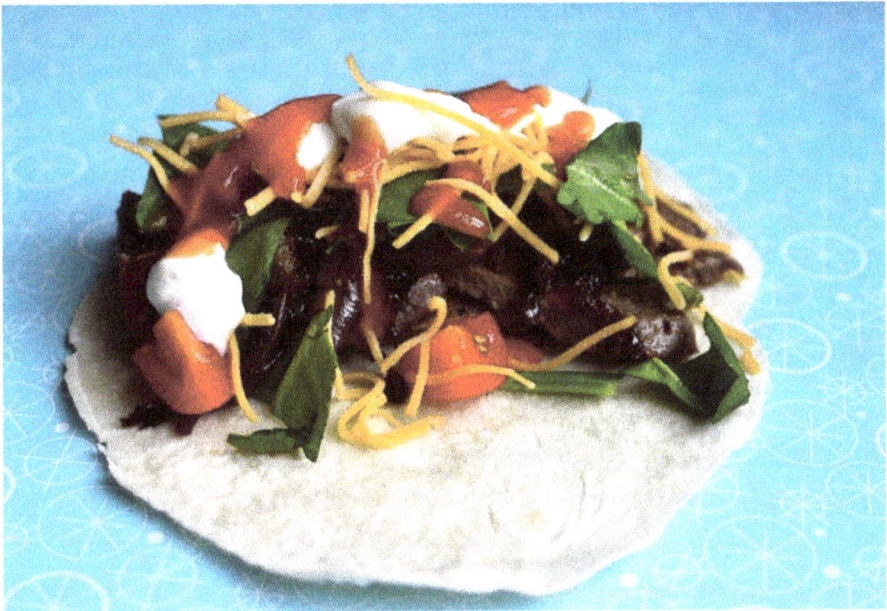

Beef Stroganoff

Servings: 4 Servings

Ingredients:

- 1½ pounds (680 g) beef round steak, cut into strips
- ½ cup (80 g) chopped onion
- 10 ounces (280 g) low-sodium cream of mushroom soup
- 8 ounces (225 g) mushrooms, sliced
- ¼ cup (60 ml) water 1 tablespoon (3 g) chives
- ½ teaspoon minced garlic
- 1 teaspoon Worcestershire sauce
- ¼ cup (60 ml) white wine
- 1 tablespoon (8 g) flour
- 16 ounces (460 g) fat-free sour cream

Directions:

1. Place the beef in the bottom of slow cooker. Place onion on top of beef and then add mushroom soup, mushrooms, and water. Season with chives, garlic, and Worcestershire sauce. In a small bowl, mix together the wine with the flour. Pour over the beef. Cover and cook on low for 6 to 7 hours. Stir in the sour cream and continue cooking for 1 hour.

Nutrition Info:

Per serving: 373 g water; 448 calories (43% from fat, 42% from protein, 15% from carb); 45 g protein; 21 g total fat; 11 g saturated fat; 6 g monounsaturated fat; 1 g polyunsaturated fat; 17 g carb; 1 g fiber; 4 g sugar; 578 mg phosphorus; 142 mg calcium; 5 mg iron; 424 mg sodium; 1299 mg potassium; 462 IU vitamin A; 115 mg ATE vitamin E; 6 mg vitamin C; 143 mg cholesterol

Beef And Eggplant

Servings: 6 Servings

Ingredients:

- 2 cups (164 g) eggplant, peeled and cubed
- 1 can (8 ounces, or 225 g) no-salt-added tomato sauce
- ½ cup (50 g) chopped celery
- ½ cup (80 g) chopped onion
- ¼ cup (38 g) chopped green pepper
- ½ teaspoon marjoram, crushed
- ¼ teaspoon cinnamon
- ¼ teaspoon nutmeg
- 1½ pounds (680 g) beef round steak, cut in 1-inch (2.5 cm) cubes

Directions:

1. In slow cooker, stir together the eggplant, tomato sauce, celery, onion, green pepper, marjoram, cinnamon, and nutmeg. Place meat on top. Cover and cook on low for 8 to 10 hours.

Nutrition Info:

Per serving: 165 g water; 173 calories (21% from fat, 64% from protein, 15% from carb); 27 g protein; 4 g total fat; 1 g saturated fat; 1 g monounsaturated fat; 0 g polyunsaturated fat; 6 g carb; 2 g fiber; 3 g sugar; 275 mg phosphorus; 20 mg calcium; 3 mg iron; 71 mg sodium; 691 mg potassium; 204 IU vitamin A; 0 mg ATE vitamin E; 12 mg vitamin C; 65 mg cholesterol

Beef With Wild Rice

Servings: 8 Servings

Ingredients:

- 1 cup (160 g) wild rice, rinsed and drained
- 1 cup (100 g) chopped celery
- 1 cup (130 g) chopped carrots
- 4 ounces (115 g) mushrooms, sliced
- 1 cup (160 g) chopped onion
- ½ cup (55 g) slivered almonds
- 2 pounds (900 g) beef round steak, cut in bite-size pieces
- 2 cups (475 ml) low-sodium beef broth

Directions:

1. Layer ingredients in slow cooker in order listed. Do not stir. Cover and cook on low 6 to 8 hours. Stir before serving.

Nutrition Info:

Per serving: 198 g water; 291 calories (27% from fat, 44% from protein, 29% from carb); 32 g protein; 9 g total fat; 2 g saturated fat; 4 g monounsaturated fat; 1 g polyunsaturated fat; 21 g carb; 3

g fiber; 3 g sugar; 412 mg phosphorus; 50 mg calcium; 3 mg iron; 118 mg sodium; 775 mg potassium; 2751 IU vitamin A; 0 mg ATE vitamin E; 3 mg vitamin C; 65 mg cholesterol

Sausage Stew

Servings: 8 Servings

Ingredients:

- 2 tablespoons (28 ml) olive oil
- 1 cup (160 g) chopped onion
- 1 pound (455 g) turkey kielbasa, thinly sliced
- 2 cans (15 ounces, or 425 g) no-salt-added great northern beans, undrained
- 2 cups (490 g) no-salt-added tomato sauce
- 4 ounces (115 g) diced green chilies
- 1 cup (130 g) thinly sliced carrots
- ½ cup (75 g) chopped green bell pepper
- ¼ teaspoon Italian seasoning
- ½ teaspoon thyme
- ¼ teaspoon black pepper

Directions:

1. Heat in oil in a large skillet over medium-high heat. Sauté onions and kielbasa until onions are soft. Transfer onions and kielbasa to slow cooker. Add all remaining ingredients to cooker and stir together well.

Cover and cook on low 8 to 10 hours or until vegetables are tender.

Nutrition Info:

Per serving: 214 g water; 320 calories (39% from fat, 20% from protein, 41% from carb); 17 g protein; 14 g total fat; 4 g saturated fat; 7 g monounsaturated fat; 2 g polyunsaturated fat; 33 g carb; 7 g fiber; 4 g sugar; 178 mg phosphorus; 82 mg calcium; 3 mg iron; 464 mg sodium; 698 mg potassium; 2944 IU vitamin A; 0 mg ATE vitamin E; 32 mg vitamin C; 40 mg cholesterol

Beef Roast With Apples

Servings: 9 Servings

Ingredients:

- 3 pounds (1 1/3 kg) beef round roast
- 1 cup (235 ml) water
- 1 teaspoon Salt-Free Seasoning Blend
- ½ teaspoon Worcestershire sauce
- ¼ teaspoon garlic powder
- 2 apples, quartered
- 1 cup (160 g) sliced onion

Directions:

1. In a large nonstick skillet coated with nonstick cooking spray, brown roast on all sides. Transfer to slow cooker. Add water to the skillet, stirring to loosen any browned bits; pour over roast. Sprinkle with seasoning blend, Worcestershire sauce, and garlic powder. Top with apple and onion. Cover and cook on low for 5 to 6 hours or until the meat is tender.

Nutrition Info:

Per serving: 177 g water; 215 calories (24% from fat, 65% from protein, 10% from carb); 34 g protein; 6 g total fat; 2 g saturated fat; 2 g monounsaturated fat; 0 g polyunsaturated fat; 5 g carb; 1 g fiber; 4 g sugar; 337 mg phosphorus; 38 mg calcium; 3 mg iron; 98 mg sodium; 601 mg potassium; 11 IU vitamin A; 0 mg ATE vitamin E; 3 mg vitamin C; 76 mg cholesterol

Mexican Beef Roast

Servings: 10 Servings

Ingredients:

- 4 pounds (1.8 kg) beef round roast
- 1 can (28 ounces, or 785 g) no-salt-added stewed tomatoes
- 2 cups (520 g) low-sodium salsa, your choice of heat
- 4 ounces (115 g) diced green chilies
- 2 small onions, cut in chunks
- 1½ cups (225 g) sliced green bell peppers

Directions:

1. Brown the roast on top and bottom in a nonstick skillet and place in slow cooker. In a bowl, combine stewed tomatoes, salsa, and green chilies. Spoon over meat. Cover and cook on low 8 to 10 hours or until the meat is tender but not dry. Add onions halfway through cooking time in order to keep fairly crisp. Push down into the sauce. One hour before serving, add pepper slices. Push down into the sauce. Remove meat from cooker and allow to rest 10 minutes before slicing.

Nutrition Info:

Per serving: 306 g water; 285 calories (22% from fat, 60% from protein, 18% from carb); 42 g protein; 7 g total fat; 2 g saturated fat; 3 g monounsaturated fat; 0 g polyunsaturated fat; 12 g carb; 3 g fiber; 7 g sugar; 439 mg phosphorus; 91 mg calcium; 5 mg iron; 271 mg sodium; 1053 mg potassium; 368 IU vitamin A; 0 mg ATE vitamin E; 31 mg vitamin C; 91 mg cholesterol

Savory Pork

Servings: About 2

Cooking Time: 9 Hrs

Ingredients:

- ½ tbsp. Extra-Virgin Olive Oil
- 1 small sliced Onion
- 8 small Potatoes
- ½ tsp. ground Black Pepper
- Pinch of Salt
- ½ tsp.Garlic Powder
- 1 tbsp.fresh Sage (rubbed)
- 1 tbsp.fresh Rosemary (crushed)
- 1 tsp. Thyme (ground)
- 2 trimmed Loin Pork Chops
- 15-ounces low-fat Mushroom Soup
- ¼ cup White Wine

Directions:

1. Place oil, potatoes and onion in the slow cooker. Sprinkle on seasoning.
2. Toss well to coat.
3. Remove fat from Pork chops.

4. Place them over the vegetables in slow cooker.

5. In a bowl, mix wine and mushroom soup well.

6. Pour the mixture over the chops.

7. Cook on "low" heat for 6 hrs.

8. Serve hot.

Nutrition Info:

(Estimated Amount Per Serving):425 Calories; 18.7 g Total Fat; 66.7 mg Cholesterol; 819.4 mg Sodium; 33.2 mg Carbohydrates; 4.7 g Dietary Fiber; 24.6 g Protein

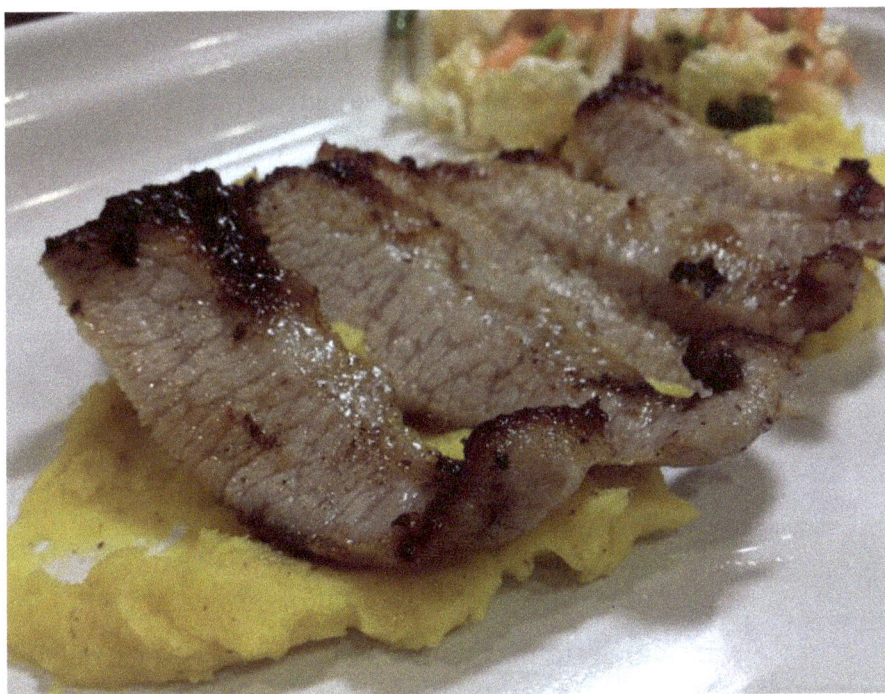

Asian Ribs

Servings: 9 Servings

Ingredients:

- ¼ cup (60 g) brown sugar
- 1 cup (235 ml) low-sodium soy sauce
- ¼ cup (60 ml) sesame oil
- 2 tablespoons (28 ml) olive oil
- 2 tablespoons (28 ml) rice vinegar
- 2 tablespoons (28 ml) lime juice
- 2 tablespoons (20 g) minced garlic
- 2 tablespoons (12 g) minced fresh ginger
- ½ teaspoon hot pepper sauce
- 3 pounds (1 1/3 kg) country-style pork ribs

Directions:

1. Stir together the brown sugar, soy sauce, sesame oil, olive oil, rice vinegar, lime juice, garlic, ginger, and hot pepper sauce in the slow cooker. Add the ribs; cover and refrigerate for 8 hours or overnight. Before cooking, drain marinade and discard. Cook on low for 9 hours.

Nutrition Info:

Per serving: 28 g water; 104 calories (78% from fat, 6% from protein, 16% from carb); 2 g protein; 9 g total fat; 1 g saturated fat; 5 g monounsaturated fat; 3 g polyunsaturated fat; 4 g carb; 0 g fiber; 1 g sugar; 37 mg phosphorus; 10 mg calcium; 1 mg iron; 92 mg sodium; 81 mg potassium; 8 IU vitamin A; 0 mg ATE vitamin E; 2 mg vitamin C; 0 mg cholesterol

Smoked Sausage And Cabbage

Servings: 4-6

Cooking Time: 10 Hrs

Ingredients:

- 1 small head Cabbage, shredded
- 1 large chopped Onion
- 1 ½ pounds Smoked Turkey Sausage
- 7 small Red Potatoes
- 1 cup Apple Juice
- 1 tbsp. Dijon Mustard
- 1 tbs. Cider Vinegar
- 2 tbsp. Brown Sugar
- 1 tsp. Caraway Seeds
- Pepper to taste

Directions:

1. In a 6 qt. cooker, place onion, cabbage & sausage in a layer.
2. Cook on high for 10 mins
3. In a bowl, whisk rest of the ingredients.
4. Now, pour this mixture on the cabbage.
5. Sprinkle on the seasonings.

6. Cook on "low" for 10 hrs.

7. Serve hot.

Nutrition Info:

(Estimated Amount Per Serving): 244.4 Calories; 10.5 g Total Fat; 75 mg Cholesterol; 945.5 mg Sodium; 18.3 mg Carbohydrates; 3.8 g Dietary Fiber; 15.5 g Protein

Southern Stuffed Pork Chops

Servings: 4 Servings

Ingredients:

- 4 pork loin chops, 1-inch (2.5 cm) thick
- 2 cups (150 g) dry corn bread stuffing mix
- 2 tablespoons (28 ml) low-sodium chicken broth
- 1/3 cup (80 ml) orange juice
- 1 tablespoon (7 g) finely chopped pecans
- ¼ cup (60 ml) light corn syrup
- ½ teaspoon grated orange peel

Directions:

1. With a sharp knife cut a horizontal slit in side of each chop, forming a pocket for stuffing. Combine stuffing with remaining ingredients. Fill pockets with stuffing. Place on metal rack in slow cooker. Cover and cook on low for 6 to 8 hours. Uncover and brush with sauce. Cook on high for 15 to 20 minutes.

Nutrition Info:

Per serving: 106 g water; 295 calories (20% from fat, 32% from protein, 48% from carb); 24 g protein; 7 g total fat; 2 g saturated

fat; 3 g monounsaturated fat; 1 g polyunsaturated fat; 35 g carb; 3 g fiber; 7 g sugar; 254 mg phosphorus; 36 mg calcium; 2 mg iron; 340 mg sodium; 471 mg potassium; 59 IU vitamin A; 2 mg ATE vitamin E; 9 mg vitamin C; 64 mg cholesterol

Salsa Beef

Servings: 6 Servings

Ingredients:

- 1 tablespoon (15 ml) olive oil
- 2 pounds (900 g) beef round steak, cut in bite-size cubes
- 2 cups (520 g) low-sodium salsa
- 1 can (8 ounces, or 225 g) no-salt-added tomato sauce
- ½ teaspoon minced garlic
- 2 tablespoons (30 g) brown sugar
- 1 cup (180 g) no-salt-added diced tomatoes

Directions:

1. Heat oil in a large skillet over medium-high heat; brown beef cubes. Place in slow cooker. Combine remaining ingredients and add to cooker. Cover and cook on low 6 to 8 hours.

Nutrition Info:

Per serving: 247 g water; 271 calories (25% from fat, 54% from protein, 20% from carb); 36 g protein; 7 g total fat; 2 g saturated fat; 4 g monounsaturated fat; 1 g polyunsaturated fat; 14 g carb; 2

g fiber; 9 g sugar; 376 mg phosphorus; 47 mg calcium; 4 mg iron; 265 mg sodium; 1036 mg potassium; 399 IU vitamin A; 0 mg ATE vitamin E; 10 mg vitamin C; 86 mg cholesterol

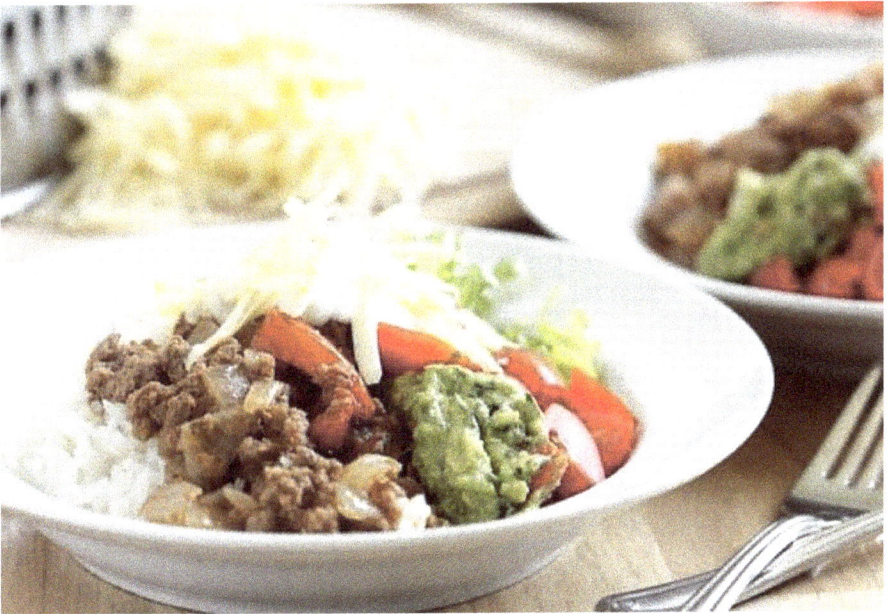

Pork Chops And White Beans

Servings: 2

Cooking Time: 4 Hrs

Ingredients:

- 1 ½ tsp. Olive Oil
- ¼ tsp. Black Pepper
- ½ diced Carrot
- ¼ cupChicken Broth (low sodium)
- ¼ tsp.Rosemary (dried)
- ¼ tsp.Kosher Salt
- 2 pork chops (boneless)
- ½ diced Yellow Onion
- 1 minced clove Garlic
- 7.5 oz. Cannellini Beans
- Chopped Parsley

Directions:

1. Season the chops with pepper and salt.
2. Sauté them in oil for 3 min on each side.
3. Transfer them to a plate.
4. In same pan, sauté rest of the ingredients except Parsley.

5. Cook for 4 mins.

6. Transfer the cooked mixture to the slow cooker along with the broth.

7. Cook on "low" for 2 hrs.

8. Add the tomatoes along with the herbs and beans.

9. Cook for 1 more hour on low.

10. Place the pork into the slow cooker.

11. Cook for 10 mins on "high".

12. Serve after garnishing with parsley.

Nutrition Info:

(Estimated Amount Per Serving): 458 Calories; 21 g Total Fats; 78 mg Cholesterol; 357 mg Sodium; 34 mg Carbohydrates; 8 g Dietary Fiber; 33 g Protein

Barbeque Beef

Servings: About 12

Cooking Time: 9 Hrs

Ingredients:

- 3 lbs Chuck Roast (boneless)
- 1 tsp. Garlic Powder
- Salt
- 1 tsp. Onion Powder
- Pepper to taste
- 18 ounces Barbeque Sauce

Directions:

1. After placing roast in the cooker, sprinkle on the seasoning.
2. Now, pour barbeque sauce over the roast.
3. Cook the roast on "low" for 8 hrs.
4. Transfer the roast to plate and shred.
5. Now, add the shredded roast back in the cooker and cook for one more hour.
6. Serve hot

Nutrition Info:

(Estimated Amount Per Serving):265.7 Calories; 4.9 g Total Fat; 81.6 mg Cholesterol; 106.8 mg Sodium; 23.9 mg Carbohydrates; 0 g Dietary Fiber; 29.0 g Protein

Barbecue Pork Roast

Servings: 8 Servings

Ingredients:

- 3 pounds (1 1/3 kg) boneless pork loin roast, cut in half
- 1 can (8 ounces, or 225 g) no-salt-added tomato sauce
- ¼ cup (60 ml) low-sodium soy sauce
- ½ cup (100 g) sugar
- 2 teaspoons dry mustard

Directions:

1. Place roast in slow cooker. Combine remaining ingredients in a bowl. Pour over roast. Cover and cook on low 6 to 8 hours or on high 3 to 4 hours until meat is tender but not dry.

Nutrition Info:

Per serving: 153 g water; 323 calories (32% from fat, 48% from protein, 20% from carb); 38 g protein; 11 g total fat; 4 g saturated fat; 5 g monounsaturated fat; 1 g polyunsaturated fat; 15 g carb; 0 g fiber; 14 g sugar; 370 mg phosphorus; 15 mg calcium; 2 mg iron;

105 mg sodium; 838 mg potassium; 111 IU vitamin A; 3 mg ATE vitamin E; 4 mg vitamin C; 94 mg cholesterol

Beef With Carrots And Turnips

Servings: About 12

Cooking Time: 8 Hrs

Ingredients:

- 1 tbsp. Kosher Salt
- 2 tsp. Cinnamon (ground)
- ½ tsp. Allspice (ground)
- ½ tsp. Pepper (ground)
- ¼ tsp. Cloves (ground)
- 3 ½ pounds Chuck Roast
- 2 tbsp. Olive Oil (extra virgin)
- 1 chopped Onion
- 3 sliced cloves Garlic
- 1 cup Red Wine
- 28 ounces whole Tomato
- 5 sliced carrots
- 2 diced Turnips
- Chopped Basil

Directions:

1. Mix all dry spices in a bowl. Season the beef with the spice mixture.

2. In a skillet, brown the beef for 5 mins in oil.

3. Remove it and place it into the slow cooker.

4. In same pan, sauté onion and garlic.

5. Add the wine and tomatoes.

6. Boil the wine mixture.

7. Transfer the wine mixture to the slow cooker.

8. Cook them on "low" for 8 hrs.

9. Serve it hot after slicing the beef.

Nutrition Info:

(Estimated Amount Per Serving): 318 Calories; 11 g Total Fat; 99 mg Cholesterol; 538 mg Sodium; 13 mg Carbohydrates; 3 g Dietary Fiber; 35 g Protein

Pot Roast In A Slow Cooker

Servings: About 6

Cooking Time: 6 Hrs

Ingredients:

- 1 chopped large, sweet Onion
- 1 cup sliced Portobello Mushrooms
- 3 lb. Beef Chuck Roast
- ½ tsp. Salt
- ¼ tsp. Pepper
- 1 cup Beef Broth or Red Wine
- 1 tbsp. Brown Sugar
- 1 tbsp. Dijon Mustard
- 1 tsp. Worcestershire Sauce
- 2 tbsp. Corn Starch

Directions:

1. Place mushrooms and onions in the slow cooker.
2. Coat roast with pepper and salt.
3. Place the roast into the slow cooker.
4. In a bowl, mix all the ingredients except cornstarch.
5. Pour the mixture into the slow cooker.
6. Cook on "low" for 6 hrs.

7. In a bowl, mix cornstarch with 2 tbsp. of water. Stir well.

8. Add the mixture to the slow cooker.

9. Cook again for 30 mins.

10. Slice beef and serve on heated plates.

Nutrition Info:

(Estimated Amount Per Serving): 382 Calories; 11 g Total Fat; 141 mg Cholesterol; 395 mg Sodium; 8 mg Carbohydrates; 1 g Dietary Fiber; 51 g Protein

Pepper Steak

Servings: About 6

Cooking Time: 9 Hrs

Ingredients:

- 1 ½ pounds boneless Beef Steaks
- 2 diced Onions
- 1 chopped clove Garlic
- ½ tsp. chopped Ginger
- ½ cup Beef Broth
- 3 tbsp. Tamari Sauce
- ¼ cup Cold Water
- 2 green and 2 red (sliced) bell peppers
- 2 sliced Tomatoes

Directions:

1. Cut the beef into 6 equal pieces.
2. In a bowl, combine ginger, tamari sauce and garlic. Marinate the beef for 2 hrs. at least.
3. In the slow cooker, spread pepper and onion on the bottom.
4. Place beef along with the marinade in the slow cooker.

5. Pour broth into the slow cooker.

6. Cook on "low" for 8 hrs.

7. Serve the beef on heated plates

Nutrition Info:

(Estimated Amount Per Serving): 349 Calories; 23 g Total Fat; 107 mg Cholesterol; 371 mg Sodium; 11 mg Carbohydrates; 2 g Dietary Fiber; 36 g Protein

Quick Stroganoff

Servings: 4 Servings

Ingredients:

- 1 pound (455 g) beef round steak, cubed
- 1 can (10 ounces, or 280 g) low-sodium cream of mushroom soup
- 1 cup (230 g) fat-free sour cream

Directions:

1. Place beef in slow cooker. Cover with mushroom soup. Cover and cook on low 8 hours or on high 4 to 5 hours. Before serving, stir in sour cream.

Nutrition Info:

Per serving: 191 g water; 263 calories (43% from fat, 44% from protein, 13% from carb); 28 g protein; 12 g total fat; 6 g saturated fat; 4 g monounsaturated fat; 1 g polyunsaturated fat; 8 g carb; 0 g fiber; 2 g sugar; 342 mg phosphorus; 76 mg calcium; 3 mg iron; 355 mg sodium; 777 mg potassium; 231 IU vitamin A; 62 mg ATE vitamin E; 1 mg vitamin C; 90 mg cholesterol

Mushroom Pot Roast

Servings: 9 Servings

Ingredients:

- 1 pound (455 g) mushrooms, sliced
- 3 pounds (1 1/3 kg) beef round roast
- 2 tablespoons (15 g) onion soup mix
- 12 ounces (355 ml) beer
- ½ teaspoon black pepper

Directions:

1. Place the mushrooms in the bottom of a slow cooker and then set the roast on top of the mushrooms. Sprinkle the onion soup mix over the beef and pour the beer over everything; season with black pepper. Cover and cook on low 9 to 10 hours or until the meat easily pulls apart with a fork.

Nutrition Info:

Per serving: 192 g water; 221 calories (25% from fat, 69% from protein, 6% from carb); 35 g protein; 6 g total fat; 2 g saturated fat; 2 g monounsaturated fat; 0 g polyunsaturated fat; 3 g carb; 1 g fiber; 1 g sugar; 377 mg phosphorus; 35 mg calcium; 3 mg iron; 98 mg sodium; 718 mg potassium; 0 IU vitamin A; 0 mg ATE vitamin E; 1 mg vitamin C; 76 mg cholesterol

Glazed Pork Roast

Servings: 12 Servings

Ingredients:

- 2 cups (475 ml) low-sodium chicken broth
- 1 cup (320 g) apricot preserves
- 1 cup (160 g) chopped onion
- 2 tablespoons (22 g) Dijon mustard
- 4 pounds (1.8 kg) boneless pork loin roast

Directions:

1. Mix broth, preserves, onion, and mustard in slow cooker. Cut pork to fit. Add to cooker. Cover and cook on low for 8 to 9 hours or high for 4 to 5 hours until done.

Nutrition Info:

Per serving: 170 g water; 313 calories (30% from fat, 44% from protein, 26% from carb); 34 g protein; 10 g total fat; 3 g saturated fat; 5 g monounsaturated fat; 1 g polyunsaturated fat; 20 g carb; 1 g fiber; 14 g sugar; 329 mg phosphorus; 19 mg calcium; 1 mg iron; 129 mg sodium; 692 mg potassium; 13 IU vitamin A; 3 mg ATE vitamin E; 4 mg vitamin C; 83 mg cholesterol

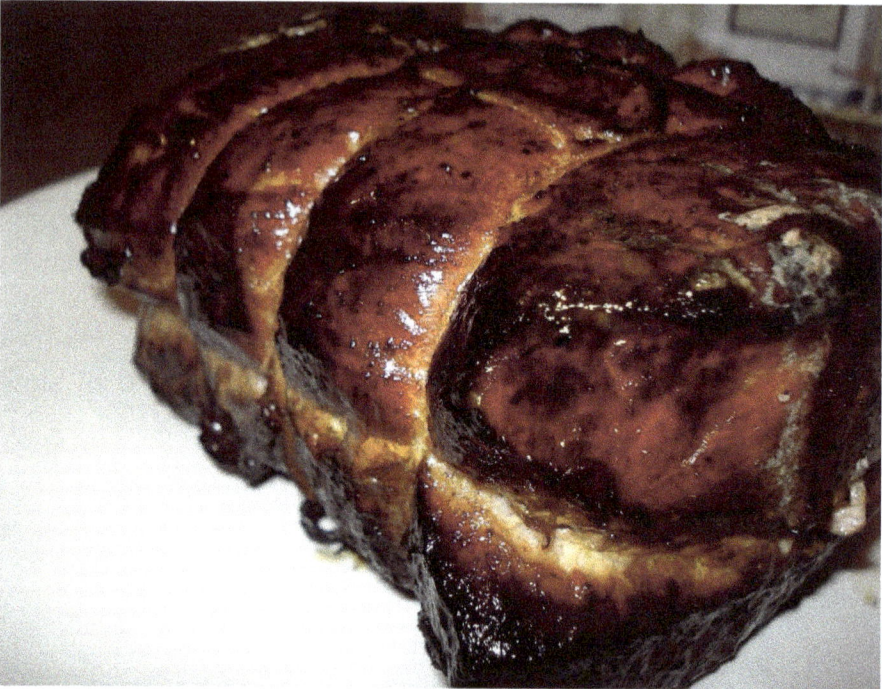

Chicken With Mushrooms

Servings: 4 Servings

Ingredients:

- 4 boneless skinless chicken breasts
- 10 ounces (280 g) low-sodium cream of mushroom soup
- 1 cup (230 g) sour cream
- 8 ounces (225 g) mushrooms, sliced
- 4 slices low-sodium bacon, cooked and crumbled

Directions:

1. Place chicken in slow cooker. In a mixing bowl, combine soup, sour cream, and mushrooms. Pour over chicken. Cover and cook on low 4 to 5 hours or until chicken is tender but not dry. Sprinkle with bacon before serving.

Nutrition Info:

Per serving: 217 g water; 252 calories (46% from fat, 38% from protein, 16% from carb); 24 g protein; 13 g total fat; 6 g saturated fat; 4 g monounsaturated fat; 1 g polyunsaturated fat; 10 g carb; 1 g fiber; 3 g sugar; 324 mg phosphorus; 83 mg calcium; 1 mg iron;

156 mg sodium; 750 mg potassium; 249 IU vitamin A; 67 mg ATE vitamin E; 3 mg vitamin C; 76 mg cholesterol

Cranberry Barbecued Turkey

Servings: 6 Servings

Ingredients:

- 3 pounds (1/3 kg) turkey legs
- 1 pound (455 g) jellied cranberry sauce
- ½ cup (140 g) chili sauce
- 2 tablespoons (28 ml) cider vinegar
- ½ teaspoon cinnamon

Directions:

1. Place turkey in slow cooker. Combine remaining ingredients and pour over turkey. Cover and cook on low for 8 to 9 hours or on high for 4 to 5 hours.

Nutrition Info:

Per serving: 143 g water; 242 calories (22% from fat, 47% from protein, 32% from carb); 28 g protein; 6 g total fat; 2 g saturated fat; 1 g monounsaturated fat; 2 g polyunsaturated fat; 19 g carb; 1 g fiber; 18 g sugar; 255 mg phosphorus; 29 mg calcium; 2 mg iron; 132 mg sodium; 409 mg potassium; 220 IU vitamin A; 0 mg ATE vitamin E; 3 mg vitamin C; 102 mg cholesterol

Sesame Chicken Thighs

Servings: 8 Servings

Ingredients:

- 3 pounds (1 1/3 kg) chicken thighs, skin removed
- 1¼ cups (425 g) honey
- 1 cup (235 ml) low-sodium soy sauce
- ½ cup (120 g) low-sodium ketchup
- 1 tablespoon (15 ml) canola oil
- 2 tablespoons (28 ml) sesame oil
- 1 teaspoon minced garlic
- ¼ cup (36 g) sesame seeds, toasted

Directions:

1. Place chicken in slow cooker. Combine remaining ingredients except sesame seeds. Pour over chicken. Cover and cook on low 5 hours or on high 2½ hours. Sprinkle sesame seeds over top just before serving.

Nutrition Info:

Per serving: 171 g water; 467 calories (27% from fat, 30% from protein, 43% from carb); 36 g protein; 14 g total fat; 3 g saturated fat; 5 g monounsaturated fat; 5 g polyunsaturated fat; 51 g carb; 1

g fiber; 47 g sugar; 357 mg phosphorus; 73 mg calcium; 3 mg iron; 252 mg sodium; 558 mg potassium; 251 IU vitamin A; 34 mg ATE vitamin E; 3 mg vitamin C; 141 mg cholesterol

Chicken And Stuffing

Servings: 12 Servings

Ingredients:

- 2½ cups (570 ml) low-sodium chicken broth
- 1 cup (225 g) unsalted butter, melted
- ¼ cup (40 g) chopped onions
- ½ cup (50 g) celery, chopped
- 4 ounces (115 g) mushrooms, sliced
- 1 tablespoon (1.3 g) parsley
- 1¼ teaspoons sage
- 1 teaspoon poultry seasoning
- ½ teaspoon pepper
- 12 cups (600 g) bread cubes
- ½ cup (120 ml) egg substitute
- 10 ounces (280 g) low-sodium cream of chicken soup
- 6 cups (840 g) cubed cooked chicken breast

Directions:

1. Combine all ingredients except bread, egg substitute, soup, and chicken in saucepan. Simmer for 10 minutes. Place bread cubes in large bowl. Combine egg substitute and soup. Stir into broth mixture until

smooth. Pour over bread and toss well. Layer half of stuffing and then half of chicken into slow cooker. Repeat layers. Cover and cook on low 4½ to 5 hours.

Nutrition Info:

Per serving: 270 g water; 422 calories (45% from fat, 27% from protein, 28% from carb); 29 g protein; 21 g total fat; 11 g saturated fat; 6 g monounsaturated fat; 2 g polyunsaturated fat; 29 g carb; 4 g fiber; 3 g sugar; 271 mg phosphorus; 106 mg calcium; 3 mg iron; 238 mg sodium; 749 mg potassium; 1171 IU vitamin A; 132 mg ATE vitamin E; 5 mg vitamin C; 101 mg cholesterol

Chicken And Broccoli Casserole

Servings: 8 Servings

Ingredients:

- 1 cup (185 g) uncooked long-grain rice
- 3 cups (700 ml) low-sodium chicken broth
- 10 ounces (280 g) low-sodium cream of chicken soup
- 2 cups (280 g) chopped cooked chicken breast
- ¼ teaspoon garlic powder
- 1 teaspoon onion powder
- 1 cup (115 g) shredded Cheddar cheese
- 1 pound (455 g) frozen broccoli, thawed

Directions:

1. Combine all ingredients except broccoli in slow cooker. Cook on high for 3 to 4 hours or on low 6 to 7 hours. One hour before end of cooking time, stir in broccoli.

Nutrition Info:

Per serving: 201 g water; 251 calories (28% from fat, 31% from protein, 41% from carb); 19 g protein; 8 g total fat; 4 g saturated fat; 2 g monounsaturated fat; 1 g polyunsaturated fat; 26 g carb;

2 g fiber; 2 g sugar; 258 mg phosphorus; 167 mg calcium; 2 mg iron; 212 mg sodium; 475 mg potassium; 528 IU vitamin A; 45 mg ATE vitamin E; 51 mg vitamin C; 48 mg cholesterol

Shredded Chicken

Servings: 12 Servings

Ingredients:

- 4 pounds (1.8 kg) chicken thighs, skinned
- 4 thyme sprigs
- 4 parsley stems
- 2 bay leaves
- ½ teaspoon garlic
- ½ teaspoon black peppercorns
- 4 cups (950 ml) low-sodium chicken broth

Directions:

1. Place chicken thighs in slow cooker. Make a bouquet garni by cutting an 8-inch (20 cm) square from a double thickness of 100-percent-cotton cheesecloth. Place thyme sprigs, parsley stems, bay leaves, garlic, and peppercorns in the center of the cheesecloth square. Bring up corners of the cheesecloth and tie with 100-percent-cotton kitchen string. Add bouquet garni to slow cooker. Pour broth over all. Cover and cook on low for 7 to 8 hours or on high for 3½ to 4 hours. Remove bouquet garni and discard. Using a slotted spoon, transfer chicken to a large bowl. When

chicken is cool enough to handle, remove meat from bones. Using two forks, shred meat. Add enough of the cooking juices to moisten meat. Strain and reserve cooking juices to use for chicken stock. Place chicken and chicken stock in separate airtight containers and refrigerate for up to 3 days or freeze for up to 3 months.

Nutrition Info:

Per serving: 189 g water; 183 calories (31% from fat, 69% from protein, 0% from carb); 30 g protein; 6 g total fat; 2 g saturated fat; 2 g monounsaturated fat; 1 g polyunsaturated fat; 0 g carb; 0 g fiber; 0 g sugar; 263 mg phosphorus; 19 mg calcium; 2 mg iron; 174 mg sodium; 374 mg potassium; 99 IU vitamin A; 30 mg ATE vitamin E; 0 mg vitamin C; 125 mg cholesterol

Sweet And Sour Chicken

Servings: 6 Servings

Ingredients:

- 3 pounds (1 1/3 kg) chicken breast halves, skinned
- ¾ cup (213 g) frozen lemonade concentrate, thawed
- 3 tablespoons (45 g) packed brown sugar
- 3 tablespoons (45 g) low-sodium ketchup
- 1 tablespoon (15 ml) vinegar
- 2 tablespoons (16 g) cornstarch
- 2 tablespoons (15 ml) cold water

Directions:

1. Place chicken in slow cooker. In a medium bowl combine lemonade, brown sugar, ketchup, and vinegar. Pour over chicken. Cover and cook on low for 6 to 7 hours or on high for 3 to 3½ hours. Transfer chicken to a serving platter; cover and keep warm. Pour cooking liquid into a medium saucepan. Skim off fat. Combine cornstarch and the water; stir into liquid in saucepan. Cook and stir over medium heat until thickened and bubbly. Cook and stir for 2 minutes more. Spoon sauce over chicken.

Nutrition Info:

Per serving: 180 g water; 484 calories (16% from fat, 60% from protein, 24% from carb); 71 g protein; 8 g total fat; 2 g saturated fat; 3 g monounsaturated fat; 2 g polyunsaturated fat; 28 g carb; 0 g fiber; 25 g sugar; 525 mg phosphorus; 44 mg calcium; 3 mg iron; 174 mg sodium; 659 mg potassium; 118 IU vitamin A; 14 mg ATE vitamin E; 8 mg vitamin C; 193 mg cholesterol

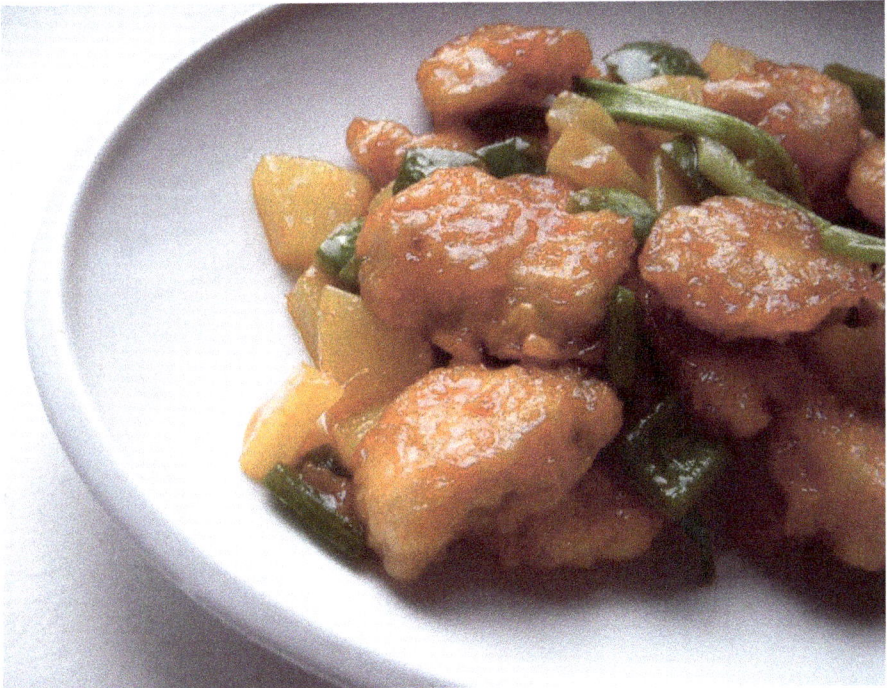

Chicken And Dumplings

Servings: 8 Servings

Ingredients:

- 4 cups (560 g) cubed cooked chicken
- 6 cups (1.4 L) low-sodium chicken broth
- 1 tablespoon (4 g) fresh parsley
- 1 cup (160 g) chopped onion
- 1 cup (100 g) chopped celery
- 6 potatoes, diced
- 12 ounces (340 g) frozen green beans
- 1 cup (130 g) sliced carrots
- For the Dumplings:
- 2 cups (250 g) flour
- 4 teaspoons (18 g) baking powder
- ¼ cup (60 ml) egg substitute
- 1 tablespoon (15 ml) olive oil
- ½ cup (120 ml) skim milk

Directions:

1. To make the soup: Combine all soup ingredients in slow cooker. Cover and cook on low 4 to 6 hours.

Transfer to a large soup kettle with lid. Bring to a boil and then reduce heat to simmer.

2.   To make the dumplings: Combine flour and baking powder in a large bowl. In a separate bowl, combine egg substitute, olive oil, and milk until smooth. Add to flour mixture and stir until combined. Drop by large tablespoons on top of simmering broth. Cover and simmer without lifting the lid for 18 minutes.

Nutrition Info:

Per serving: 550 g water; 441 calories (10% from fat, 22% from protein, 68% from carb); 24 g protein; 5 g total fat; 1 g saturated fat; 2 g monounsaturated fat; 1 g polyunsaturated fat; 76 g carb; 8 g fiber; 6 g sugar; 428 mg phosphorus; 239 mg calcium; 5 mg iron; 457 mg sodium; 1736 mg potassium; 3188 IU vitamin A; 18 mg ATE vitamin E; 36 mg vitamin C; 40 mg cholesterol

Chicken Cacciatore

Servings: 5 Servings

Ingredients:

- 1½ cups (240 g) sliced onions
- 3 pounds (1/3 kg) chicken thighs, skin removed
- ½ teaspoon minced garlic
- 1 can (14 ounces, or 400 g) no-salt-added stewed tomatoes
- 1 cup (245 g) no-salt-added tomato sauce
- ½ teaspoon pepper
- ½ teaspoon oregano
- ½ teaspoon basil
- 1 bay leaf
- ½ cup (120 ml) dry white wine

Directions:

1. Place onions in bottom of slow cooker. Lay chicken over onions. Combine remaining ingredients and pour over chicken. Cover and cook on low 6 to 6½ hours. Remove bay leaf before serving.

Nutrition Info:

Per serving: 383 g water; 401 calories (26% from fat, 59% from protein, 15% from carb); 55 g protein; 11 g total fat; 3 g saturated fat; 3 g monounsaturated fat; 3 g polyunsaturated fat; 14 g carb; 2 g fiber; 8 g sugar; 507 mg phosphorus; 77 mg calcium; 4 mg iron; 248 mg sodium; 1054 mg potassium; 497 IU vitamin A; 54 mg ATE vitamin E; 16 mg vitamin C; 226 mg cholesterol

Cassoulet

Servings: 6 Servings

Ingredients:

- 1¼ cups (228 g) dried navy beans
- 4 cups (950 ml) water
- 2 tablespoons (28 ml) olive oil
- 3 pounds (1 1/3 kg) chicken, cut up
- ½ cup (65 g) finely chopped carrot
- ½ cup (50 g) chopped celery
- ½ cup (80 g) chopped onion
- 1½ cups (355 ml) low-sodium tomato juice
- 1 tablespoon (15 ml) Worcestershire sauce
- ½ teaspoon basil
- ½ teaspoon oregano
- ½ teaspoon paprika

Directions:

1. In large saucepan, bring beans and 4 cups (950 ml) water to boiling. Reduce heat and simmer, covered, for 1½ hours. Pour beans and liquid into bowl. Heat oil in a large skillet over medium-high heat and brown the chicken. In slow cooker, place chicken, carrot, celery,

and onion. Drain beans; mix with tomato juice, Worcestershire sauce, basil, oregano, and paprika. Pour over meat mixture. Cover and cook on low for 8 hours. Remove chicken and mash bean mixture slightly, if desired.

Nutrition Info:

Per serving: 282 g water; 347 calories (20% from fat, 62% from protein, 18% from carb); 52 g protein; 7 g total fat; 2 g saturated fat; 2 g monounsaturated fat; 2 g polyunsaturated fat; 16 g carb; 5 g fiber; 4 g sugar; 471 mg phosphorus; 72 mg calcium; 4 mg iron; 220 mg sodium; 909 mg potassium; 2338 IU vitamin A; 36 mg ATE vitamin E; 23 mg vitamin C; 159 mg cholesterol

Texas Chicken

Servings: 8 Servings

Ingredients:

- 1 cup (185 g) uncooked long-grain rice
- 1 can (28 ounces, or 785 g) no-salt-added diced tomatoes
- 1 can (6 ounces, or 170 g) no-salt-added tomato paste
- 3 cups (700 ml) water
- 2 tablespoons (15 g) Salt-Free Mexican Seasoning
- 4 boneless skinless chicken breasts, cut into 1-inch (2.5 cm) cubes
- 1½ cups (240 g) chopped onions
- 1 cup (150 g) chopped green bell pepper
- 4 ounces (115 g) diced green chilies
- 1 teaspoon garlic powder
- ¼ teaspoon pepper

Directions:

1. Combine all ingredients in large slow cooker. Cover and cook on low 4 to 4½ hours or until rice is tender and chicken is cooked.

Nutrition Info:

Per serving: 285 g water; 178 calories (5% from fat, 27% from protein, 69% from carb); 12 g protein; 1 g total fat; 0 g saturated fat; 0 g monounsaturated fat; 0 g polyunsaturated fat; 31 g carb; 3 g fiber; 7 g sugar; 148 mg phosphorus; 66 mg calcium; 3 mg iron; 119 mg sodium; 617 mg potassium; 538 IU vitamin A; 2 mg ATE vitamin E; 37 mg vitamin C; 21 mg cholesterol

Cranberry-orange Turkey Breast

Servings: 9 Servings

Ingredients:

- ¼ cup (80 g) orange marmalade
- 1 pound (455 g) whole berry cranberry sauce
- 2 teaspoons (8 g) orange peel, grated
- 3 pounds (1/3 kg) turkey breast

Directions:

1. Combine marmalade, cranberries, and peel in a bowl. Place the turkey breast in the slow cooker and pour half the orange- cranberry mixture over the turkey. Cover and cook on low 7 to 8 hours or on high 3½ to 4 hours until turkey juices run clear. Add remaining half of orange-cranberry mixture for the last half hour of cooking. Remove turkey to warm platter and allow to rest for 15 minutes before slicing. Serve with orange-cranberry sauce.

Nutrition Info:

Per serving: 145 g water; 272 calories (8% from fat, 53% from protein, 38% from carb); 36 g protein; 2 g total fat; 1 g saturated

fat; 0 g monounsaturated fat; 1 g polyunsaturated fat; 26 g carb; 1 g fiber; 24 g sugar; 312 mg phosphorus; 24 mg calcium; 2 mg iron; 115 mg sodium; 478 mg potassium; 29 IU vitamin A; 0 mg ATE vitamin E; 2 mg vitamin C; 91 mg cholesterol

4-WEEK MEAL PLAN

Week 1

Monday
Breakfast: Tofu Frittata
Lunch: Pork Chops In Beer
Dinner: Stewed Tomatoes

Tuesday
Breakfast: Tapioca
Lunch: Creamy Beef Burgundy
Dinner: Oregano Salad

Wednesday
Breakfast: Fruit Oats
Lunch: Smothered Steak
Dinner: Black Beans With Corn Kernels

Thursday
Breakfast: Grapefruit Mix
Lunch: Pork For Sandwiches
Dinner: Stuffed Acorn Squash

Friday
Breakfast: Berry Yogurt
Lunch: Cranberry Pork Roast

Dinner: Greek Eggplant

Saturday
Breakfast: Soft Pudding
Lunch: Pan-asian Pot Roast
Dinner: Thyme Sweet Potatoes

Sunday
Breakfast: Black Beans Salad
Lunch: Short Ribs
Dinner: Barley Vegetable Soup

Week 2

Monday
Breakfast: Carrot Pudding
Lunch: French Dip
Dinner: Butter Corn

Tuesday
Breakfast: Apple Cake
Lunch: Italian Roast With Vegetables
Dinner: Orange Glazed Carrots

Wednesday
Breakfast: Almond Milk Barley Cereals
Lunch: Honey Mustard Ribs
Dinner: Cinnamon Acorn Squash

Thursday

Breakfast: Cashews Cake

Lunch: Pizza Casserole

Dinner: Glazed Root Vegetables

Friday

Breakfast: Artichoke Frittata

Lunch: Hawaiian Pork Roast

Dinner: Stir Fried Steak, Shiitake And Asparagus

Saturday

Breakfast: Mexican Eggs

Lunch: Apple Cranberry Pork Roast

Dinner: Cilantro Brussel Sprouts

Sunday

Breakfast: Stewed Peach

Lunch: Swiss Steak

Dinner: Italian Zucchini

Week 3

Monday

Breakfast: Lamb Cassoule t

Lunch: Glazed Pork Roast

Dinner: Cilantro Parsnip Chunks

Tuesday

Breakfast: Fruited Tapioca

Lunch: Swiss Steak In Wine Sauce

Dinner: Corn Casserole

Wednesday

Breakfast: Baby Spinach Shrimp Salad

Lunch: Italian Pork Chops

Dinner: Pilaf With Bella Mushrooms

Thursday

Breakfast: Coconut And Fruit Cake

Lunch: Italian Pot Roast

Dinner: Italian Style Yellow Squash

Friday

Breakfast: Apple And Squash Bowls

Lunch: Beef With Horseradish Sauce

Dinner: Stevia Peas With Marjoram

Saturday

Breakfast: Slow Cooker Chocolate Cake

Lunch: Oriental Pot Roast

Dinner: Broccoli Rice Casserole

Sunday

Breakfast: Fish Omelet

Lunch: Barbecued Ribs

Dinner: Italians Style Mushroom Mix

Week 4

Monday
Breakfast: Brown Cake
Lunch: Ham And Scalloped Pota toes
Dinner: Broccoli Casserole

Tuesday
Breakfast: Stevia And Walnuts Cut Oats
Lunch: Pork And Pineapple Roast

Wednesday
Breakfast: Walnut And Cinnamon Oatmeal
Lunch: Barbecued Brisket
Dinner: Dinner: Slow Cooker Lasagna

Thursday
Breakfast: Tender Rosemary Sweet Potatoes
Lunch: Barbecued Short Ribs
Dinner: Brussels Sprouts Casserole

Friday
Breakfast: Orange And Maple Syrup Quinoa
Lunch: Beer-braised Short Ribs
Dinner: Pasta And Mushrooms

Saturday
Breakfast: Vanilla And Nutmeg Oatmeal
Lunch: Lamb Stew
Dinner: Onion Cabbage

Sunday

Breakfast: Pecans Cake

Lunch: Barbecued Ham

Dinner: Cheese Broccoli

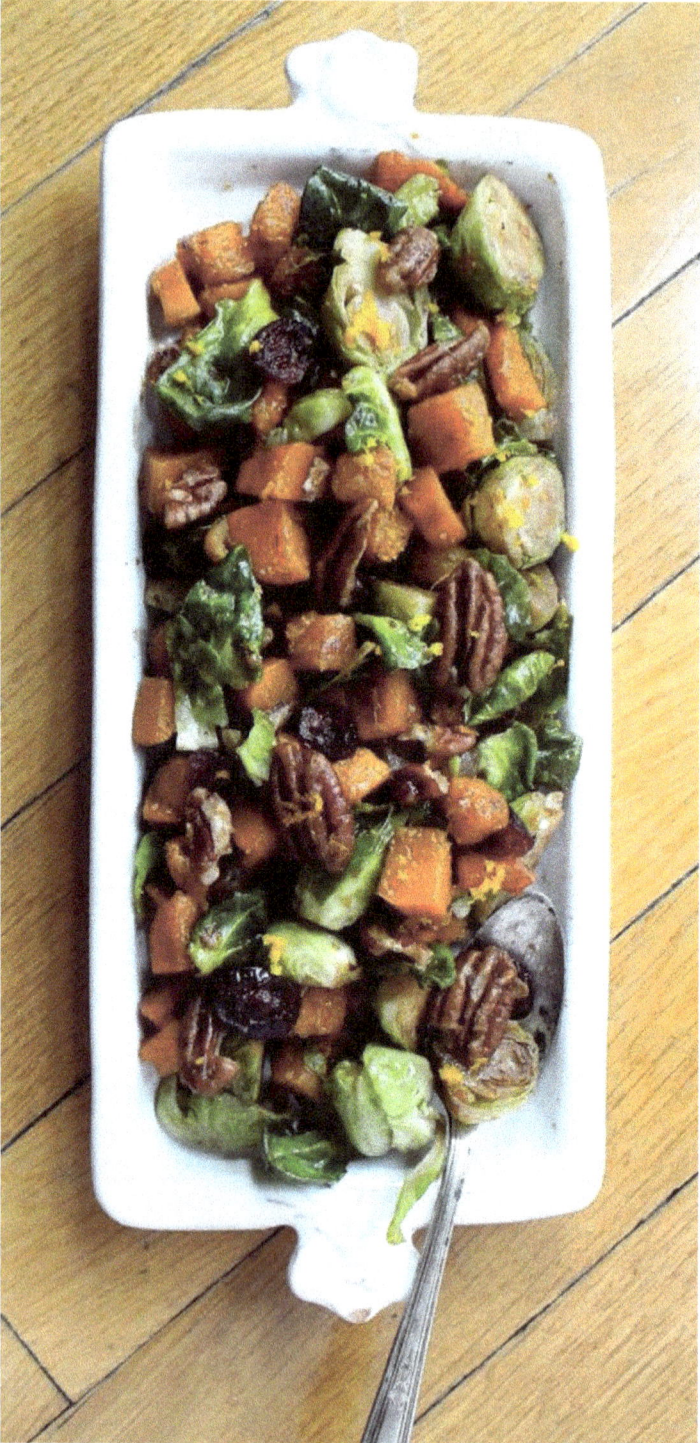

www.ingramcontent.com/pod-product-compliance
Lightning Source LLC
Chambersburg PA
CBHW050752030426
42336CB00012B/1783